INTRODUCTION

This book is about understanding your body type and achieving a healthy lifestyle. We'll explore the science behind body fat. And promote long-term Achievement.

Everything mentioned in this book is interconnected kindly pay attention for better results

if you feel stuck in between or have any question related to weight loss or need any guidance feel free to contact.

FOLLOW US ON INSTAGRAM- RV_07
GMAIL - jaidevandson@gmail.com

CAHPTER'S

The Body Type's

These are three body types described by psychologist William H. O Sheldon in the 1940s.

Ectomorph: Lean and slender with low body fat and muscle mass. With a thin appearance, narrow shoulders, and hips, they often have high metabolic rates. Their bones are lighter

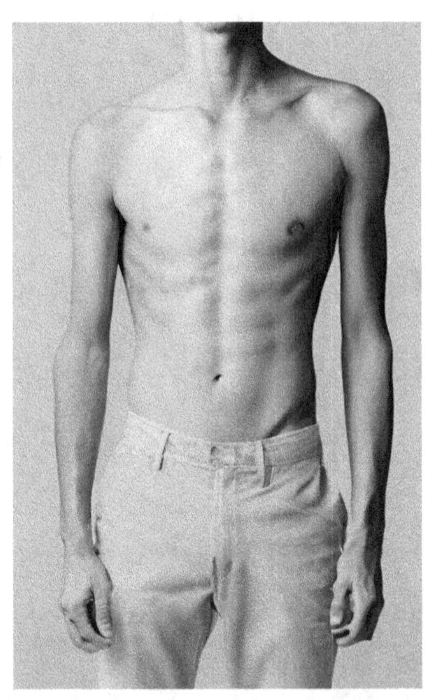

and less dense compared to others, which can make it challenging for them to gain weight and muscle mass.

Mesomorph: Athletic and muscular with a strong build. Mesomorphs have a rectangular-shaped body with broad shoulders and a narrow waist. That makes it easier for them to gain and lose weight and have well-defined muscles. They have a balanced metabolism, It allows them to build muscle quickly. Due to their natural muscularity, mesomorphs often excel in sports and physical activities.

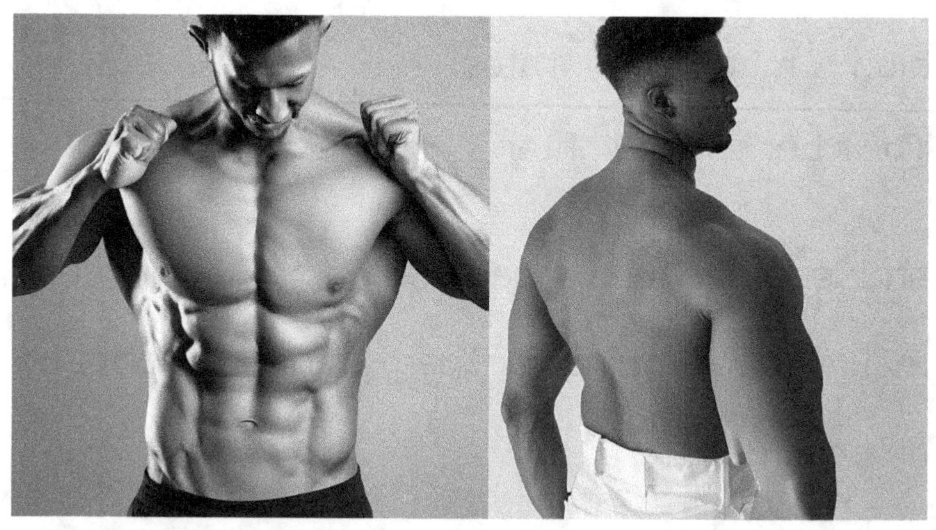

Endomorph: Rounded and soft with a higher percentage of body fat. Endomorphs often have a round or pear-shaped body with a wider waist and hips. They tend to have more body fat, which makes it challenging to achieve a lean physique. Endomorphs often have a slower metabolic rate, which means they will struggle more to lose body fat.

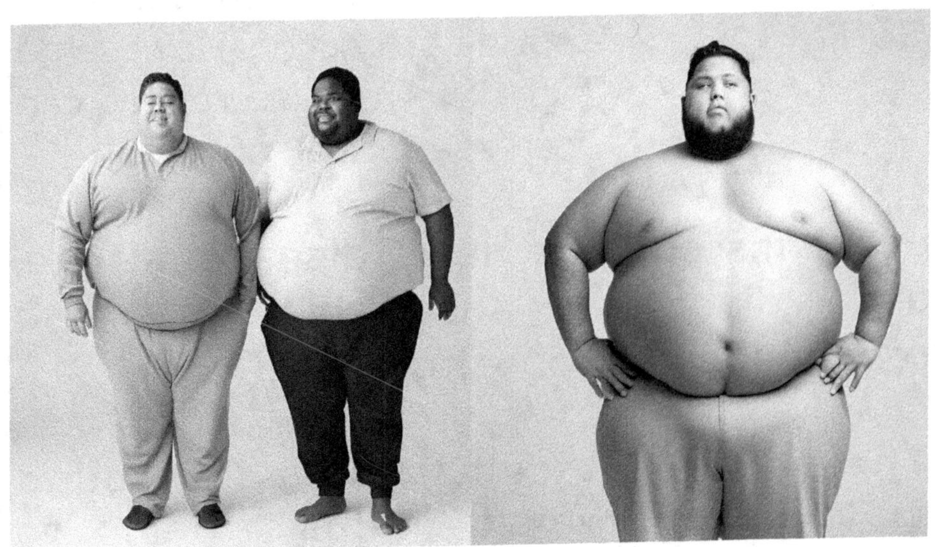

The Body Fat

There are three fat in our body white fat, brown fat, and beige fat.

The white fat is located under the skin acts as energy storage and releases energy when needed.

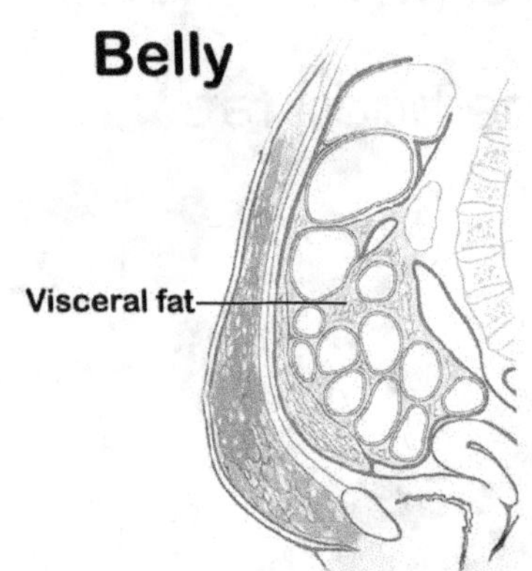

Belly

Visceral fat surrounds the organs in the abdomen to provide protection. However, a high level of visceral fat can .increase the risk of health problems such as heart disease, stroke, and diabetes, and this is also responsible for obesity

The brown fat cell is typically found in babies, which helps them to regulate body temperature by burning calories.

How does the environment (Surrounding temperature) impact body metabolism

The impact of surrounding temperature on body metabolism is significant. Hot and cold temperatures can affect digestion differently for different individuals due to various factors.
Here are some important considerations:

When it's hot, the body works hard to regulate its temperature. Digesting non-vegetarian food requires more energy and time compared to digesting carbohydrates or fats. In hot temperatures, this added metabolic load from digesting meat may further strain the body's resources.

Digestive enzymes play an essential function in breaking down food in the gut. Cold weather can slightly decrease the activity of these enzymes, further impacting digestion. During colder months, people often crave and consume richer, heavier foods. These foods, typically higher in fat and calories, take longer to digest than lighter, fiber-rich options. Eat smaller meals instead of large, heavy ones. This can ease the workload on your digestive system.

Vegetables are generally lighter on the stomach and easier to digest than protein-rich foods like meat. They contain fiber, which promotes regular bowel movements and supports gut health

Non-vegetarian foods are rich in protein, and protein digestion requires adequate hydration to support the breakdown and absorption of amino acids. In hot weather, increased sweating and fluid loss can lead to dehydration, which can impair digestive processes, including protein digestion.

Many vegetables have high water content, which helps maintain hydration levels in hot weather. Proper hydration is also important for digestion and absorbing nutrition. Additionally, vegetables are rich in essential vitamins, minerals, and antioxidants that support overall health and digestion.

Avoid red meat as much as possible Challenges for Digestion

Red meat is high in fat, especially fatty cuts, and higher in fat content than other protein sources like chicken or fish. Fat takes longer to digest than protein or carbohydrates, which can slow down the digestive process and potentially lead to bloating or discomfort.

Red meat is generally low in fiber, a crucial component for digestive health and regularity

It's not preferable when you are on a mission to reduce body fat but if you want to eat. Balance your red meat intake with plenty of fiber-rich vegetables and whole grains to aid digestion. Drink water sufficiently to support your gut.

How Fat Effects on Body

When we get overweight fat cells can cause plaque build-up in the arteries (atherosclerosis). This plaque narrows the arteries and restricts blood flow to vital organs. leads to high blood pressure eventually weakening the heart muscle which contributes to chronic inflammation throughout the body. This inflammation can damage blood vessels.

Reason for having body fat

Low muscle mass, continuous sitting, eating more than needed, eating too many sweet things, carbonated drinks, junk food, smoking, drinking alcohol, overeating red meat, low activity, less sleep, stress, etc.

Overcome body fat

To reduce overall body fat you need to change your daily routine step by step follow instructions below.

Diet plan

Step one is changing your diet plan. Don't worry. It sounds typical, but it's not as difficult as you think. First, we need to increase water intake to flush out unwanted toxins and keep kidneys and liver keeps you healthy. It also helps purify the blood and hydrate your body. Within 24 hours, drinking water intake should be 4 liters of fluid for men and 3 liters for women.

Second increased antioxidants act as scavengers, neutralizing free radicals and preventing them from causing harm. This helps reduce oxidative stress, a condition caused by an imbalance between free radicals and antioxidants in the body. Some antioxidants possess anti-inflammatory properties, potentially reducing chronic inflammation linked to several health issues.

Here is a list of antioxidants Fruits:

Fruits:

- **Rich in Vitamin C:** Oranges, grapefruits, kiwifruit, strawberries, guava, papaya
- **High in Anthocyanins (beneficial for eye health):** Blueberries, blackberries, raspberries, cranberries, cherries, red grapes

- **Rich in Carotenoids (vitamin A precursors):** Mangoes, cantaloupe, peaches, apricots

Vegetables:

- **Cruciferous Vegetables:** Broccoli, Brussels sprouts, kale, cauliflower (rich in sulforaphane)
- **Dark Leafy Greens:** Spinach, kale, collard greens (high in various antioxidants)
- **Bell Peppers:** Red, orange, yellow (abundant in vitamin C and carotenoids)
- **Artichokes:** A good source of cynarin, a potential antioxidant

Whole Grains:

- **Whole Wheat Bread and Brown Rice:** Contain fiber and ferulic acid, an antioxidant
- **Oats:** Rich in beta-glucan fiber with antioxidant properties

Nuts and Seeds:

- **Almonds, Walnuts, Pecans:** Provide vitamin E and other antioxidants
- **Chia Seeds and Flaxseeds:** Good sources of omega-3 fatty acids and antioxidants

Other Foods:

- **Dark Chocolate (choose 70% cocoa or higher):** Contains flavanols, beneficial antioxidants
- **Green Tea:** Rich in epigallocatechin gallate
- **Tomatoes:** Contain lycopene, an antioxidant linked to heart health

High fibrous food in diet

Improved Digestion and Gut Health: Fiber adds bulk to your stool and helps it move smoothly through your digestive system, preventing constipation. Prebiotic benefits soluble fiber acts as a prebiotic, feeding the good bacteria in your gut microbiome. These bacteria contribute to a healthy digestive system.

Fiber helps you feel fuller for longer, potentially reducing calorie intake and aiding in weight management. Fiber can help regulate blood sugar levels by slowing down the absorption of sugar into the bloodstream.

Cruciferous Vegetables:

- **Broccoli:** 1 cup cooked: 5.6 grams fiber
- **Brussels sprouts:** 1 cup cooked: 3.8 grams fiber
- **Cauliflower:** 1 cup cooked: 2.5 grams fiber

Leafy Greens:

- **Kale:** 1 cup cooked: 5.3 grams fiber
- **Spinach:** 1 cup cooked: 4.3 grams fiber
- **Swiss Chard:** 1 cup cooked: 4.1 grams fiber

Other Vegetables:

- **Artichokes:** 1 medium artichoke: 6.9 grams fiber
- **Beets:** 1 cup cooked: 3.8 grams fiber (including beet greens)
- **Carrots:** 1 cup raw: 3.6 grams fiber

- **Sweet Potatoes:** 1 medium baked potato with skin: 4 grams of fiber
- **Green Peas: 1 cup cooked:** 8.8 grams fiber (considered a starchy vegetable)
- **Okra: 1 cup cooked:** 3.2 grams fiber
- **Asparagus: 1 cup cooked:** 2.7 grams fiber

Additional Tips:

- **Include the skin:** Whenever possible, eat the skin of vegetables, as it often contains a significant amount of fiber.
- **Cooking methods:** Steaming, roasting, or lightly stir-frying vegetables helps preserve their fiber content.
- **Variety is a Key:** Include a diverse range of high-fiber vegetables in your diet to benefit from a variety of nutrients and fiber types.

Here are some bonus high-fiber vegetables, though they may be less common in some regions:

- **Bitter Gourd: 1 cup cooked:** 7 grams fiber
- **Jicama: 1 cup chopped:** 6.4 grams fiber
- **Sweet Potatoes:** 1 medium baked potato with skin: 4 grams of fiber
- **Green Peas: 1 cup cooked:** 8.8 grams fiber (considered a starchy vegetable)
- **Okra: 1 cup cooked:** 3.2 grams fiber

Asparagus: 1 cup cooked: 2.7 grams fiber

Avoid sugar

Here is why you should avoid sugar or stop taking sugary food.

When you consume sugar, your blood glucose levels rise, provoking the pancreas to release insulin to help cells absorb glucose for energy. However, high levels of insulin also promote fat storage. Sugary foods affect hormones that regulate hunger and satiety. For instance, consuming sugar leads to rapid spikes and drops in blood sugar levels, which may increase cravings and overall food intake. This results in consuming more calories than needed when you eat large amounts of sugar, particularly fructose (found in high-fructose corn syrup), which is processed by the liver. Excessive fructose can lead to increased fat production in the liver, contributing to fat accumulation, especially in the abdominal area. High sugar intake interferes with the body's ability to oxidize fat efficiently. Instead of burning fat for energy, the body may prioritize using glucose. Which leads to an increased propensity to store fat. **Note : if you have diabetes (Sugar) please consult your Doctor.**

Lean protein food to the diet

Protein keeps you fuller for longer, potentially reducing calorie intake throughout the day. This can help manage hunger and cravings while dieting. During weight loss, some muscle loss can occur. Protein helps preserve muscle mass, which is important for metabolism and overall health. Muscle burns more calories than fat, so maintaining muscle mass can help boost your metabolism and aid in weight loss. Digesting protein has a higher thermic effect compared to fat or carbohydrates. This means your body burns more calories during protein digestion.

Lean Protein Sources:

- **Chicken breast:** A classic lean protein source, low in fat and calories.

- **Fish:** Excellent source of protein and healthy omega-3 fatty acids. Choose options like salmon, tuna, sardines, or cod.

- **Turkey breast:** Similar to chicken breast, but with a slightly different flavour profile.

- **Lentils and beans:** A plant-based protein source rich in fiber, keeping you feeling full for longer.

Start walking around with 100 to 200 hundred footsteps and then increase to 50 footsteps each day for 2 weeks in the morning and before bedtime. After 2 weeks, start running 1 km a day, then after 2 days, increase the distance.

Split your meal in half. For example, if you eat 2 pieces of bread and 2 eggs in the morning, then split it in half. After eating one-half portions, take a break for around 1 or 1/30 hours then eat the remaining half. Always remember before or after to take a gap of 20 minutes for water drinking because our body produces heat to break down food. When you drink water just after or before a meal, the temperature difference in the stomach slows down the digestion process.

For those who have low immunity and feel low energy levels in the wake time, make herbal tea with a combination of squeezed half a lemon and one teaspoon of honey, pour it into green tea, mix it well, and drink it with breakfast.

Muscle mass

Muscle mass plays a significant role in our body's immune function, digestion, and fat metabolism. It's important to understand that. How the immune system behaves in weight gain and loss.

When our daily physical activity is low, our body may dilute muscle mass to reduce the load or to save energy from unnecessary consumption of muscle and start storing it in the form of fat deposits. As a result, the body's energy requirements decrease due to the lower muscle mass. For instance, a person who works out at the gym might need 4 eggs the entire day for energy, which is directly related to muscle mass. If this person starts eating 6 eggs a day, but the body only needs 4 for energy, the excess 2 eggs are converted into fat and stored.

Build muscle mass to reduce fat

To reduce fat, focus on building muscle mass. Engage in muscle training exercises such as weight lifting, which should fatigue or stress your muscles. Before starting, ensure that you stay hydrated and monitor your breathing to ensure it feels regular. Additionally, stretch exercises help regulate blood circulation and blood pressure before weight training exercises.

Begin with a small weight, such as 10 kg, to build strength or stamina, aiming for one set of 10 repetitions. Then, gradually increase the number of repetitions each day for a week before progressing to a higher weight, such as 20 kg, while maintaining the same number of sets and reps.

Bicep curls

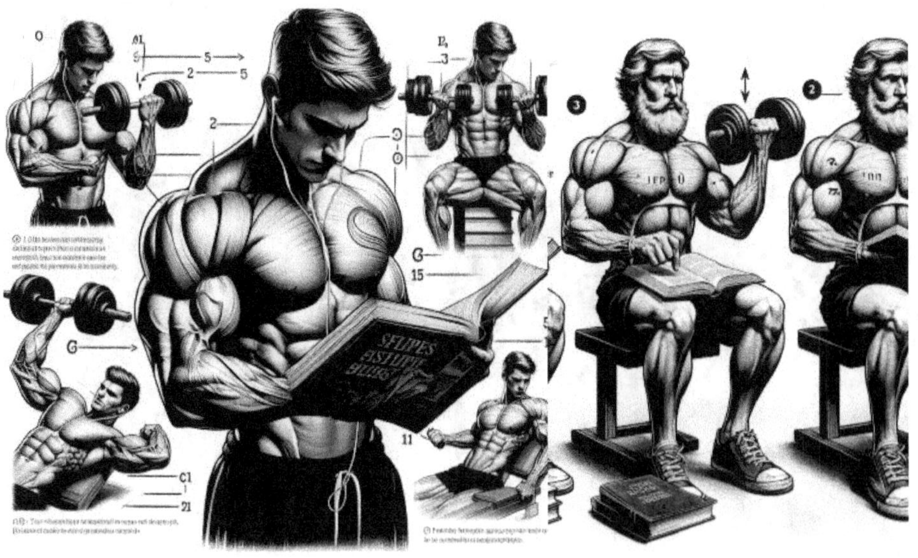

Triceps extensions

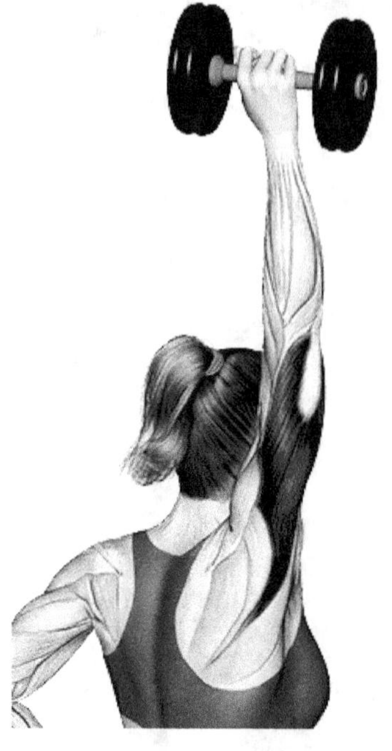

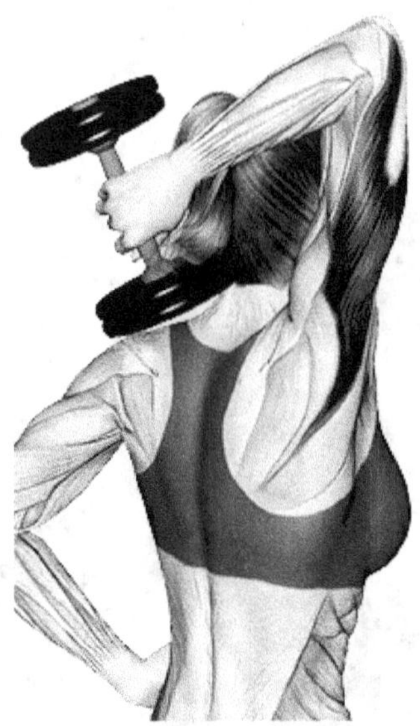

Leg extensions

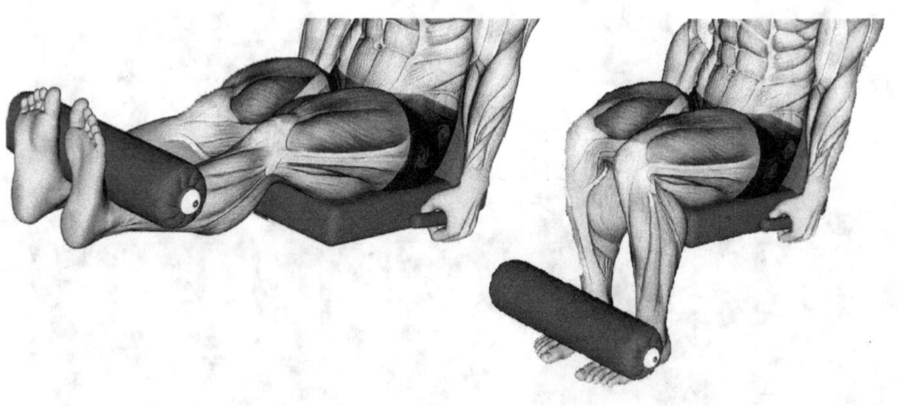

Hamstring curls

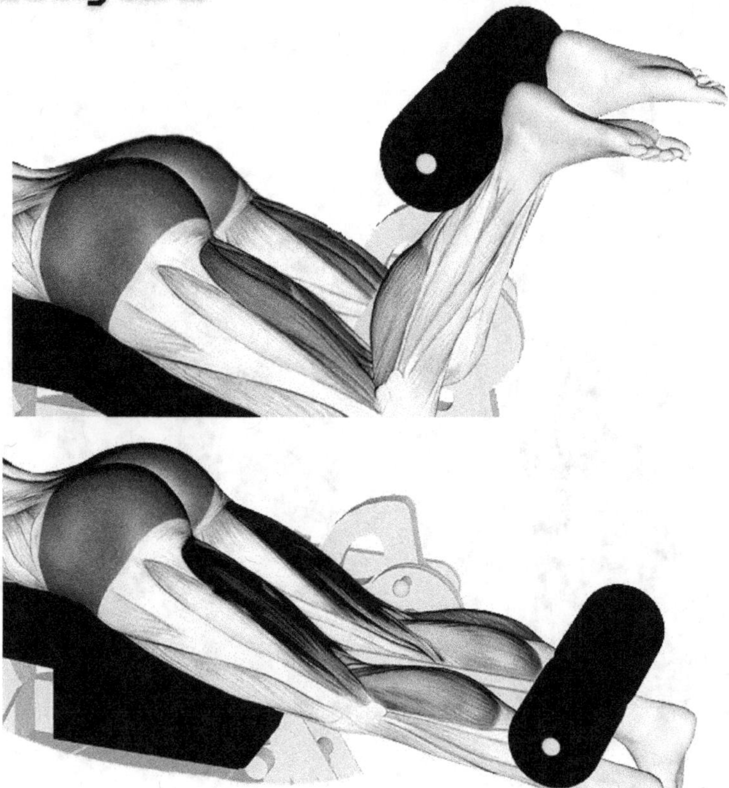

Chest press, Bench press, Shoulders press,

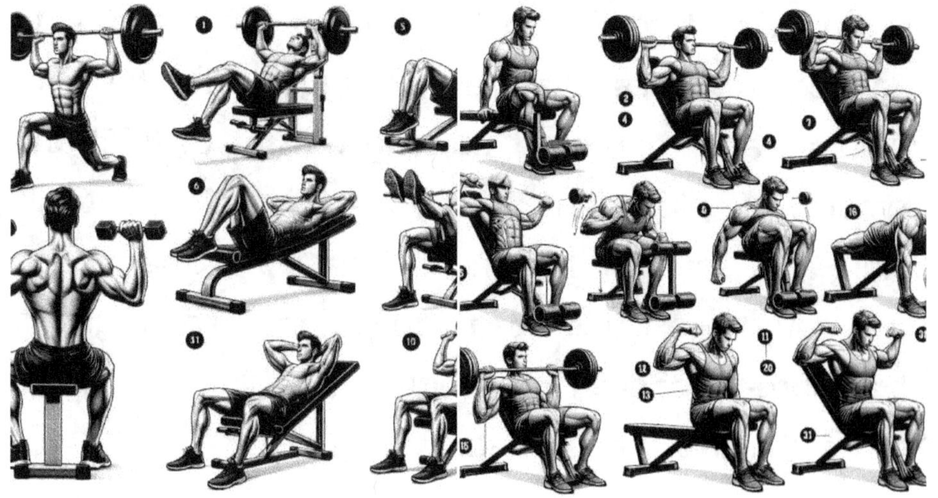

Intermediate fasting

Intermediate fasting is an eating pattern. The cycles of eating and fasting focus on when you eat rather than what you eat. Unlike traditional calorie restriction diets, it offers flexibility for those who struggle with strict dietary plans.

Here are some points about intermediate fasting:

Intermediate fasting is a cycle between eating and fasting time. The most popular method is 16/8 hour. (Fasting at night for 16 hours and eating in a day within an 8-hour) or the 5:2 days method (eating for 5 Days and restricting calories on 2 Non-consecutive days).

During fasting periods, your body undergoes a metabolic switch. Insulin levels drop, which prompts the body to access stored energy in the form of glycogen and then start burning the fat to fulfill the demand for glycogen. This process is called ketosis. While it is safe for healthy adults, it's crucial if you have any pre-existing health conditions, are pregnant, or are breastfeeding. You should consult your doctor before starting intermediate fasting.

Eating Phase

Eating Phase (8 hours): Remember to focus on nutrient-rich whole foods to provide your body with the essential vitamins, minerals, and fiber. Here's a sample breakdown of your eating.

Break fat, Lunch: Prioritize lean protein with complex carbohydrates for sustained energy. Examples are grilled chicken or fish with brown rice and roasted vegetables, a lentil soup with whole-wheat bread, or a tofu scramble with whole-wheat toast and avocado.

Snack (Optional): Choose a healthy snack to curb hunger, with fruit like berries or apples with a handful of almonds, greek yogurt with berries and chia seeds, or carrot sticks with hummus.

Dinner: A balanced plate with protein, healthy fats, and vegetables. Examples include baked salmon with roasted Brussels sprouts and quinoa, lentil stew with whole-grain bread, or a turkey stir-fry with brown rice and mixed vegetables.

General Tips:

Hydration is Key: Drink plenty of water throughout the day, especially during your fasting Phase, to support bodily functions.

Nutrient Density Matters: Choose whole foods rich in vitamins, minerals, and fiber to ensure proper nutrition during your eating.

Mindset Matters: Be patient and focus on making sustainable changes. Celebrate your progress and view intermediate fasting as a journey towards a healthier lifestyle.

Supplements vs. natural diet

Natural Diet: When you consume natural foods, they often contain fiber, which aids digestion and helps regulate bowel movement. Foods contain natural enzymes that help break down proteins, carbohydrates, and fats. They also provide a variety of vitamins, minerals, and phytonutrients that supplements cannot fill.

Supplements: Supplements are concentrated doses of specific nutrients like vitamins, minerals, and amino acids that bypass the natural processes of digestion and don't have their own natural enzymes, making them easier to absorb. Supplements are mainly in powder or pills that lack fiber and don't contribute to digestive health compared to natural food. Which is crucial for overall digestive health.

Impact on the Digestive System

Natural Diet: natural foods support a healthy digestive system by providing fiber, supporting gut microbiota diversity, and ensuring a steady release of nutrients.

Supplements: While supplements can be beneficial for addressing specific deficiencies or health conditions, relying heavily on supplements can sometimes bypass the natural process of digestion and nutrient extraction that are important for overall digestive health.

We suggest you go with a natural diet to gain long-term effects and maintain a healthy life. This information is gathered from the personal s experience of the people and information available by the professionals.

The weight loss weekly diet planner is given below. There is a cutting bleed line given above the table for cut and paste for your convivence.

Weight Loss Diet Planner Table:

	Goals	Meal Plan	Exercise	Hydration	Notes
Monday	- Calorie deficit of 500 calories	Breakfast: Whole grain cereal with skim milk	Morning: 30 mins cardio	8 glasses of water	- Prepare lunch in advance
	- Track food intake with app	Lunch: Grilled chicken salad with olive oil dressing	Afternoon: 15 mins stretching	Herbal tea or infused water	- Avoid late-night snacks
	- Drink 8 glasses of water	Snack: Greek yogurt with berries	Evening: 20 mins strength training		
Tuesday	- Include vegetables in every meal	Breakfast: Oatmeal with fruits	Morning: 30 mins brisk walk	8 glasses of water	- Plan meals for the rest of the week
	- Limit refined sugars and processed foods	Lunch: Quinoa with mixed vegetables	Afternoon: Yoga or Pilates	Herbal tea or infused water	- Focus on portion sizes
	- Evening snack: Fruit or nuts	Snack: Hummus with carrot sticks	Evening: Rest day or light activity		
Wednesday	- Achieve 10,000 steps	Breakfast: Whole grain toast with avocado	Morning: 30 mins cycling	8 glasses of water	- Check weight progress
	- Cook dinner at home	Lunch: Grilled fish with steamed broccoli	Afternoon: 15 mins core exercises	Herbal tea or infused water	- Review weekly goals
	- No eating after 8 PM	Snack: Cottage cheese with pineapple	Evening: 20 mins cardio		
Thursday	- Try a new healthy recipe	Breakfast: Smoothie with spinach, banana, and almond milk	Morning: 30 mins HIIT workout	8 glasses of water	- Reflect on challenges faced
	- Plan meals for the weekend	Lunch: Turkey wrap with whole grain tortilla	Afternoon: Stretching or flexibility exercises	Herbal tea or infused water	- Set goals for next week

Weight Loss Diet Planner Table:

	- Focus on mindful eating	Snack: Mixed nuts and dried fruits	Evening: Active rest day		
Friday	- Relax and unwind	Breakfast: Scrambled eggs with vegetables	Morning: 30 mins walk	8 glasses of water	- Celebrate small victories
	- Avoid excessive alcohol	Lunch: Lentil soup with whole grain bread	Afternoon: 15 mins yoga	Herbal tea or infused water	- Plan for the weekend
	- Plan active social activities	Snack: Fresh fruit salad	Evening: Light activity or stretching		
Saturday	- Plan for a healthy brunch	Breakfast: Whole wheat pancakes with berries	Morning: 30 mins jog or run	8 glasses of water	- Enjoy a balanced weekend
	- Grocery shopping for next week	Lunch: Grilled vegetables with quinoa	Afternoon: Active outdoor activity	Herbal tea or infused water	- Prepare for upcoming week
	- Try a new exercise class	Snack: Greek yogurt with honey and nuts	Evening: Relaxation and stretching		
Sunday	- Meal prep for the week	Breakfast: Avocado toast with poached egg	Morning: Rest day or gentle stretching	8 glasses of water	- Reflect on progress made
	- Plan active family time	Lunch: Chicken stir-fry with brown rice	Afternoon: Light yoga or meditation	Herbal tea or infused water	- Set new goals for the upcoming week
	- Evaluate weekly progress	Snack: Smoothie with protein powder	Evening: Prepare for the week ahead		

Weight Loss Tracking Table

Tips for Using the Table:

- **Date:** Enter the date of each weigh-in or measurement.
- **Weight (lbs):** Record your weight in pounds.
- **BMI:** Calculate and record your BMI (Body Mass Index) if desired.
- **Waist (in):** Optionally, track waist circumference or other body measurements.
- **Notes/Comments:** Use this column to add any relevant information such as changes in diet, exercise routine, how you feel, or any challenges faced.

BMI calculated using the following formula:

$$BMI = Height\ (m)2\ /Weight\ (kg)$$

However, if you prefer to use pounds and inches:

$$BMI = [Height\ (in)2/Weight\ (lbs)] \times 703$$

Here's a step-by-step guide to calculate BMI:

Convert Weight to Kilograms (if using pounds):If your weight is in pounds (lbs), divide it by 2.205 to convert it to kilograms (kg).

Convert Height to Meters (if using inches): If your height is in inches (in), divide it by 39.37 to convert it to meters (m).

Square the Height: Multiply the height in meters (or converted value from inches to meters) by itself (square it).

Calculate BMI: Divide the weight in kilograms by the squared height in meters (or the squared value from inches converted to meters). Or, multiply the weight in pounds by 703, then divide by the squared height in inches.

Example Calculation:

Let's say:

- Weight = 150 lbs
- Height = 5 feet 6 inches (or 66 inches)

Convert Height to Meters:

o 66 inches = 66 / 39.37 = 1.676 meters (approximately).

Square the Height:

o 1.6762=2.8071.676^2 = 2.8071.6762=2.807 square meters.

Calculate BMI:

o BMI = (150 lbs / (66 inches)^2) x 703

o BMI = (150 / 4356) x 703

o BMI   24.1

Therefore, the BMI is approximately 24.1, which falls within the normal weight range (18.5 – 24.9).

Interpretation of BMI:

- **Underweight:** BMI less than 18.5
- **Normal weight:** BMI 18.5 – 24.9
- **Overweight:** BMI 25 – 29.9
- **Obese:** BMI 30 or greater

Weight Loss Weekly Tracking Table

Date	Weight (lbs)	BMI	Waist (in)	Notes/Comments

Weight Loss Weekly Tracking Table

Date	Weight (lbs)	BMI	Waist (in)	Notes/Comments

Weight Loss Weekly Tracking Table

Date	Weight (lbs)	BMI	Waist (in)	Notes/Comments

Weight Loss Weekly Tracking Table

Date	Weight (lbs)	BMI	Waist (in)	Notes/Comments

Weight Loss Weekly Tracking Table

Date	Weight (lbs)	BMI	Waist (in)	Notes/Comments

Weight Loss Weekly Tracking Table

Date	Weight (lbs)	BMI	Waist (in)	Notes/Comments

Weight Loss Weekly Tracking Table

Date	Weight (lbs)	BMI	Waist (in)	Notes/Comments